a morning cup of tai chi ™

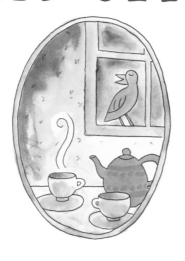

The publisher and author cannot be held responsible for injury, mishap, or damages incurred during the performance of the exercises in this book. The author recommends consultation with a healthcare professional before beginning this or any other exercise program.

"A Morning Cup of" is a trademark of Crane Hill Publishers, Inc.

Excerpt from Aldous Huxley's *Island* reprinted with permission from Harper and Row

Published by Crane Hill Publishers
www.cranehill.com

Printed in Canada

  Library of Congress Cataloging-in-Publication Data

Bright-Fey, John A.
  A morning cup of tai chi : one 15-minute routine to nurture your body, mind, and spirit / by John A. Bright-Fey.
      p. cm.
  ISBN 1-57587-220-X (alk. paper)
  1. Tai chi. I. Title.
  GV504.B76 2004
  613.7'148--dc22

                              2004004028

www.cranehill.com

10   9   8   7   6   5   4   3   2   1

a morning cup of tai chi

one 15-minute routine to nurture
your body, mind, and spirit

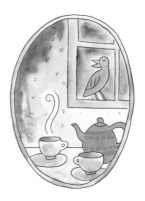

john a. bright-fey

CRANE HILL
PUBLISHERS

Acknowledgments

I'd like to thank the following individuals for their invaluable help and advice. This Morning Cup would surely not taste as sweet without their assistance:

To the faculty and student body of the Blue Dragon Academy who keep the campfires blazing in the New Forest;

To Ellen, Allison, and all the staff at Crane Hill Publishers for presenting me with this glorious opportunity;

To Charles Fechter, life-long friend and Boswell, for his continuing support during the writing and illustration process;

To Beau Gustafson of Big Swede Incorporated for his excellent pre-illustrative photographs;

To Ernie Eldredge and Tim Rocks for bringing the movements of New Forest Tai Chi to life in wonderful watercolor illustrations;

To all of you, much love and many thanks.

JB-F

This book is dedicated to my lovely wife, Kim,
who plays Tai Chi
with me

Contents

from Island *by Aldous Huxley (Harper & Row, 1962)*

"Don't imagine," Mrs. Narayan resumed, "That this is the only kind of dancing we teach. Redirecting the power generated by bad feelings is important. But equally important is directing good feelings and right knowledge into expression. Expressive movements, in this case, expressive gesture. If you had come yesterday, when our visiting master was here, I could have shown you how we teach that kind of dancing. Not today unfortunately. He won't be here again before Tuesday."

"What sort of dancing does he teach?"

Mrs. Narayan tried to describe it. No leaps, no high kicks, no running. The feet always firmly on the ground. Just bending and sideways motions of the knees and hips. All expression confined to the arms, wrists and hands, to the neck and head, to the face and, above all, the eyes. Movement from the shoulders upwards and outwards—movement intrinsically beautiful and at the same time charged with symbolic meaning. Thought taking shape in ritual and stylized gesture. The whole body transformed into a hieroglyph, a succession of hieroglyphs, of attitudes modulating from significance to significance like a poem or a piece of music. Movements of the muscles representing movements of Consciousness, the passage of Suchness into the many, of the many into the imminent and ever-present One.

"It's meditation in action," she concluded. "It's the metaphysics of the Mahayana expressed, not in words, but through symbolic movements and gestures."

Foreword

For the first time, the magic of Tai Chi is readily available to you. The book you hold in your hands is a key to true health. According to medical research, Tai Chi can improve your balance, boost your immune system, lower your blood pressure, and reduce your chronic aches and pains. As a physical therapist, I have seen it work—many times!

A Morning Cup of Tai Chi introduces you to a revolutionary style of Tai Chi that is easy to learn and fun to do. It is revolutionary because it seems to break all the rules. Unlike other books on Tai Chi, you won't find any reference to a "Stork Spreading Its Wings" or a "Snake Creeping Down." You won't be asked to memorize a complicated movement sequence.

John Bright-Fey recognized that the imagery and movements of traditional Tai Chi were too complex for the average person. His mission was to make the health benefits of Tai Chi available to everyone. He wanted to create a style of Tai Chi that anyone could do, and he did.

New Forest® Tai Chi is simply fantastic! Follow John along as he teaches you the essence of Tai Chi movement. Follow your breath as you move slowly, gracefully. Gently focus your attention and imagination. You will discover the magic for yourself! You can do THIS Tai Chi.

Kim Bright-Fey
Physical Therapist

The Beauty of Tai Chi

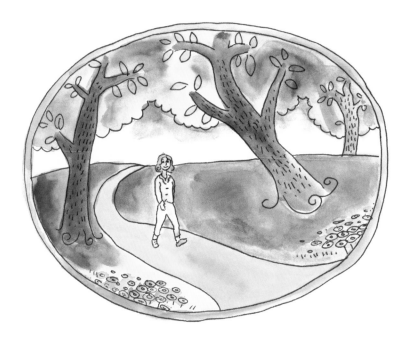

I want to share a really big secret with you. With this secret, you will be able to increase the breadth and depth of your day-to-day existence. It will almost be like you've added an extra fifty, sixty, or more years to your normal life span. Food will taste better, music will sound sweeter, and the touch of a human hand will take on a quality that will be, in a word, amazing. Along the way, you'll learn to relax, banish stress, build strength, gain flexibility, and improve your balance. Simply put, you'll start to feel great! And with practice, everyday life will get bigger, brighter, funnier, and more interesting and exciting. And what, you may ask, is your investment for this fountain of youth? You have to play for fifteen minutes a day. That's right: I said, "play." In the time it would take you to sit down and have a cup of tea or coffee, you can reconnect with yourself and get back in touch with who you really are.

The secret I want to share with you is the art of Tai Chi. Pronounced "Tie Chee," this art form is a dance of life that nurtures your body, awakens your mind, and lifts your spirits. Tai Chi first entered my life over forty years ago, and since that day, it has been my constant companion. It has seen me through great tragedy and serious illness. With it, I've felt God's heart beating next to my own, comforting me in the knowledge that we are not alone and that we never have been. Tai Chi constantly shows me new ways to embrace life and the lives that I encounter. Most importantly, my art shows me new ways to love. Now, with this Morning Cup, you can begin to experience all of this for yourself.

I've divided this book into roughly three parts. The first part will be a brief introduction to Tai Chi and its basic principles. The second part is a presentation of the Tai Chi routine itself. Most people think that there is a mountain of theory that must be learned before you can really play Tai Chi. This is simply not the case. I'll explain the absolute least you need to know about Tai Chi and then we'll get down to business and "play." The style and approach to Tai Chi we will use for our Morning Cup is the New Forest® style. This is my signature approach to the art that makes the many benefits and wonders of Tai Chi immediately available to you. I've used these methods with my students for more than a quarter of a century with marvelous results.

The third part of this book will contain more detailed information about your new art, information that I trust you will find both useful and interesting. But remember that Tai Chi is a moving physical activity that can only be explored by physically moving.

When you opened this book you entered a school without walls populated by a student body that stretches around the world. The subjects taught revolve around relaxation, playfulness, and creativity. And while most schools have a whole list of rules that you must follow, this school has only one. Rule # 1: FUN! Let's get ready to play Tai Chi.

John Bright-Fey
Birmingham, Alabama
Spring 2004

What Is Tai Chi?

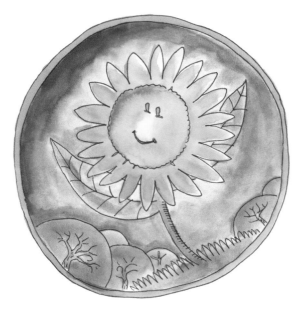

Merriam-Webster defines Tai Chi as "an ancient Chinese discipline of the meditative movements practiced as a system of exercises." It is a bodymind discipline. I use the word "bodymind" because the ancient players of Tai Chi used their discipline to bring their bodies and minds back together whenever they felt fragmented and separated from their thoughts, their lives, and the world around them. It worked so well that they elevated Tai Chi from a discipline to high art. It became physical movement poetry, a breathing exercise, moving meditation, a dynamic system of physical and intellectual conditioning, and a whole lot more. It's easy to spot people playing Tai Chi. Alone or in groups, it is usually performed deliberately, mindfully, and most often, slowly. In fact, as a child I just called it "slow motion under water," because that's the way it looked and felt. As I got older, I learned that the slow and deliberate manner of execution increased my levels of focus and concentration. It allowed me to be more present in the moment, to control pain, to sleep better, and to generally feel great!

While Tai Chi is an incredible tool for cultivating health and wellness, it has a marvelous multidimensional character and can be almost anything you want it to be. It has the power to enhance any life that it meets; that is, any life that is willing to play a little.

Real Tai Chi people don't often use words like "work out," "train," or "exercise" to describe what they do. They say "play" instead. Lewis Carroll, the Victorian author of the classics *Alice in Wonderland* and *Jabberwocky*, created a word that describes the kind of play Tai Chi people engage in. His word is "galumphing," and it represents the activity of a child's game where the rules are few, but the pretend adventures are many. This is the kind of game we all used to play one time in our life, but generally don't any more. A child is galumphing when a fallen stick becomes Excalibur and where a kitchen broom turns into a fiery horse.

As children, we played so we could explore the world around us, and in the process learn about our inner selves as well. When we played as children, we were refreshed, challenged, inquisitive, carefree, and happy. Play was an integral part of our health, growth, and development. But as we grow up, the games get more serious and responsibilities become more adult. Our minds become less adventurous and our bodies, well, they just don't work like they did when we were kids. Consequently, we stop exploring our deeper selves. It also becomes harder and harder to learn from our inner self, and when our heart speaks, we can barely hear it.

The only way to reclaim our minds, bodies, and our spirits is to learn to play again. Don't you think we could all stand to play a little every morning before we go out to meet the challenges of our day? That's precisely what the ancient creators of Tai Chi thought, and their wisdom was so profound that it survives actively and vitally to the present day.

People who cannot do typical kinds of exercise can do Tai Chi. Even if you are confined to a wheelchair, you can still be a Tai Chi player. In the land of Tai Chi, you are only as limited as your imagination. Think of it as a bottomless Morning Cup. Would you like a refill?

New Forest® Tai Chi

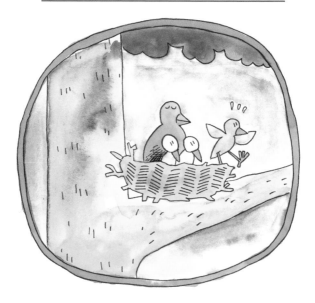

At its simplest, New Forest Tai Chi consists of deliberate and comfortable stepping while you use your hands to slowly paint imaginary shapes in the air on an invisible artist's canvas in front of you. The first kind of shape you will paint will be number shapes, specifically the numerals one through ten.

1 2 3 4 5
6 7 8 9 10

When you paint these numbers, you will imagine something specific for each of them. These are called Internal Adjustments. You will learn more about these shortly.

The second kind of shape you will paint on your imaginary canvas is the ancient Tai Chi diagram.

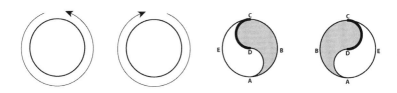

It is from this shape that the whole art of Tai Chi gets its name. The Tai Chi diagram provides a fertile field for creative movement that gently exercises your muscles and loosens your joints. You can get lost as you gently oscillate through the diagram, painting it in long, smooth, continuous strokes. As you move, you test your physical limits while imaginatively reaching out to touch your environment. Painting the diagram will also begin putting you in touch with your whole bodymind as your waist twists gently and your weight shifts gradually from one foot to the other.

If you can naturally walk forward and backward and stand still, then you can do Tai Chi stepping. Even if you can only imagine yourself walking, you can still play Tai Chi. Most of the details regarding Tai Chi stepping will be explained in the routine that follows, so there's no need to worry about them now. What is important is that you do your best to step as deliberately and mindfully as possible using whatever stride is the most balanced and comfortable for you. This is a hallmark of the New Forest approach. Every step and gesture you perform is fully adaptable. Feel free to shorten, lengthen, or otherwise change any of the movements to fit your own physical gifts and deficits.

Learning the Tai Chi routine that follows is a reasonably straightforward experience. The emphasis on natural movement and familiar shapes makes our Tai Chi easy to learn and fun to do. This style of Tai Chi is purposefully open and flexible so you can change and adjust the postures as you see fit. You are in control.

With both the number shapes and the Tai Chi diagram shapes, you have to decide what size they will be. They can be big numbers, for example, two to three feet tall—or small numbers that are only a few inches high. The same is true of your Tai Chi diagrams: big or small, you decide. Likewise, the Tai Chi steps you take can be big steps or small ones, whatever you can do, whatever you feel comfortable with. This is very important. You have to be comfortable with any Tai Chi movement you make. If, for example, your shoulder hurts when you make a big number, then paint it smaller so your shoulder doesn't hurt. Exercise of any kind can feel uncomfortable from time to time, but it's your job to adapt your Tai Chi postures to fit yourself so that you get the benefits of the exercise without excessive discomfort.

Tai Chi Breath

Many Tai Chi teachers love Chinese calligraphy. I'm no exception. The flowing lines created by brush and ink remind us of our Tai Chi movements. One of the basic tenets of Chinese brushwriting centers around the coordination of breath with the act of painting. Essentially, the calligrapher gently inhales as he prepares to write a character, and then exhales as the brush is put to paper. The breath then gently guides the brush. Whether you are painting a flower, bug, or a Chinese word, how you breathe is considered to be very important. Not only does it affect the beauty of whatever you paint, it also relaxes your body, clears your mind, and enlivens your senses.

The breath carries a special human signal with it that fixes whatever you are painting in emotional space and time. Said another way, it makes whatever you paint, write, or draw more real, more authentic. I believe it allows a portion of your soul to express itself in whatever you paint. Breath coordinated with motion is so important to Chinese painters and calligraphers that we call it the "Artist's Breath of Life" or the "Poet's Breath." We will use the same kind of breathing when we play our Tai Chi. It will allow us to get deeply inside each of our postures so the movements and their internal adjustments can work their magic on our bodyminds.

Simple Tai Chi Breathing

This will be very easy. Whenever you lift your hands in preparation to paint your number, breathe in. Then put your hands to the imaginary canvas and breathe out as you paint the number shape. Remember: imagine that your arms, hands, and fingers are really giant paintbrushes connected to an endless supply of paint or ink hidden deep inside you. Try to complete the number shape at the same time you complete your exhalation.

When playing Tai Chi, ask yourself to move and breathe slowly, but don't force your breath to be slower than is comfortable. Let the natural speed of your breathing tell you how fast to move. The bodymind has great wisdom if we will only listen to it.

For Tai Chi beginners, it is not always necessary to coordinate the breath with the movements. But it is something that you should shoot for as you become more experienced. If coordinating your breathing with your movements is confusing, or if your breathing is impaired in any way, just breathe naturally as you move slowly and deliberately through the routine. It's that simple. As you become a more experienced Tai Chi player, your breathing will naturally relax and deepen on its own. Then you can match up your movements and your breath.

The Inner Landscape of Tai Chi

Tai Chi is sometimes called the Nei Chia (pronounced "Nay CHEE-ah"), which means "esoteric, inner, or hidden exercise." This is because so much of what gives Tai Chi its unique character and artistic flavor takes place deep inside your bodymind. Simply performing slow rote movement in a regulated manner is not the authentic Tai Chi way. The shapes that you make with your hands and arms must be meaningful if they are to transform you.

I first began using number shapes in childhood to help remember the complex movements of archaic Tai Chi. I would twist and bend the numbers in my head so that I'd have a way to easily translate old Chinese postures into a form I could remember. After all, to an American child, the Chinese postures weren't culturally relevant. They came from Chinese dance, art, and philosophy. They, simply put, were not meaningful to me. But the number shapes gave me a basic structure to relate to. Eventually, I could use the 1 through 10 number shapes so familiar in our culture to explain any Tai Chi posture or movement, no matter how detailed or complicated. It allowed me to get deeply inside the movements.

As I worked to master Chinese art, poetry, movement, and philosophy, I also created mnemonics and rhyming games to help me comprehend their depths. Again, I used numbers to connect the internal secrets and philosophical roots of each posture to its physicality. I also used these games to bring poetry and music to a physically expressive level.

Now, as a teacher, I use the same number shapes and memory games to help my students. They find that the Tai Chi shapes are much easier to learn this way. More importantly, the meaning and purpose of these shapes become almost instantly accessible—just as they did for me decades earlier.

The number shapes themselves are so familiar that you should have no trouble at all following the Tai Chi routine. But if you are to truly get in touch with yourself, you need to learn the New Forest Tai Chi "1 Through 10" Game.

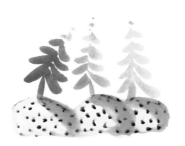

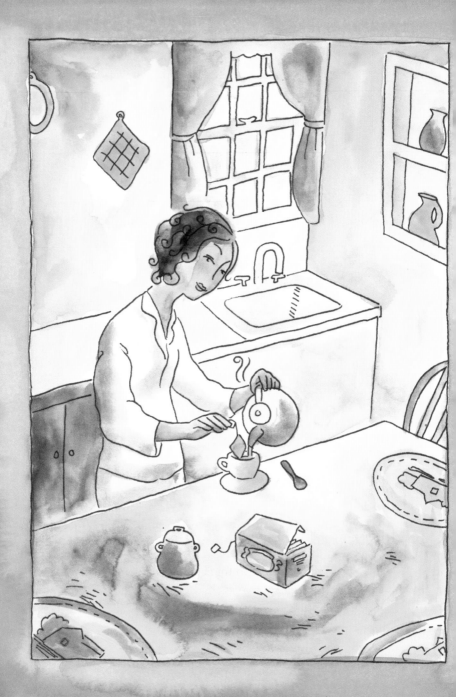

The New Forest "1 through 10" Game

If you can count from one to ten, you can play Tai Chi. It's as easy as that. The New Forest "1 through 10" keywords will introduce you to the inner landscape of Tai Chi. Start by reading the following list aloud several times.

Number	Keyword
One	FUN
Two	SHOE
Three	TREE
Four	CORE
Five	ALIVE
Six	THICK
Seven	HEAVEN
Eight	GATE
Nine	SHINE
Ten	SPIN

Now, close your eyes and count from one through ten, saying the numbers and their keywords from memory. Recite silently or aloud; you choose. If you get stuck, open your eyes and read the list again until you know all of the keywords and their associated numbers. It won't be long before you have them easily memorized. Each keyword tells you what to think about when you paint its number on your imaginary canvas.

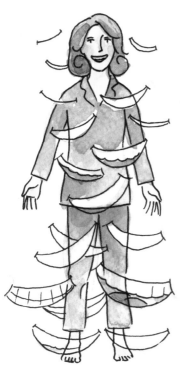

1-Fun

Think of fun. Smile gently and suggest to yourself to relax all over. You can even think of something funny! Enjoy the moment.

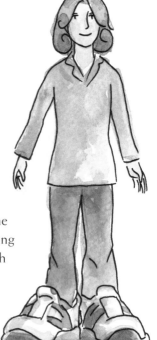

2-Shoe

Think about your toes, feet, and the shoes you're usually wearing standing firmly on the ground. Feel the earth beneath your feet.

3- Tree

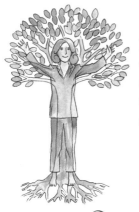

Imagine you are a huge healthy tree with massive branches full of leaves and roots penetrating deeply into the soil. You are rooted, vibrant, and stable.

4- Core

Imagine that you have a fire hydrant buried deep inside your abdomen. This hydrant, located roughly three and a half inches below your navel and inward toward the center of your body, is the place where you gather strength. It is your point of focus.

5- Alive

Pretend that pressurized life-giving water from your Four-Core is rushing out of your arms and legs at an incredible rate of speed. It's as if your arms and legs are high-pressure fire hoses and your hands and feet are the nozzles.

6-Thick

Pretend that all of the air around you is thick and viscous. It's so thick, in fact, you can feel it squishing through your fingers as you move. Imagine that if you relaxed completely, the thick air would cradle you and keep you from falling.

7-Heaven

Gently stretch up with the top of your head toward the heavens as if you were a marionette. Pretend you are being lifted subtly upward, rising above the noise and confusion of the moment. Think about something that is important to you: family, friends, religion, your goals and higher ideals.

8-Gate

Imagine that each pore of your skin is in reality a tiny gate. As you inhale, these gates swing open and draw air into them, into your bodymind. When you exhale, pretend that the gates close shut and all the life-giving energy from the air around you now circulates freely throughout your entire bodymind.

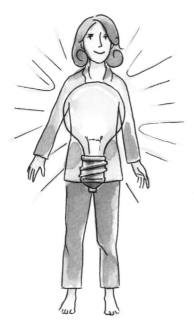

9-Shine

Imagine you're a light bulb. That's right: a giant you-shaped light bulb. As you inhale, your light is dim, but you gradually shine out brighter and brighter as you exhale. You are glowing with high-wattage brilliance.

10-Spin

Let the first nine numbers and their associated images float through your mind in any order. If one pops up in your mind with more clarity than the other, focus on it briefly, and then let it slip away until another comes up. Just let the numbers swirl and spin in your imagination.

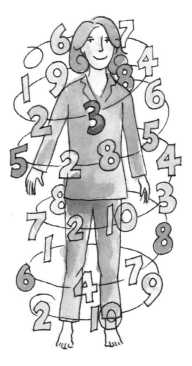

Although you'll be thinking about the One through Ten internal adjustments when you paint your Tai Chi shapes, you can think about them any time you see a number or a group of numbers. Remember you are using these visualizations to adjust your internal landscape so you can have a greater experience of the outside world. And who among us couldn't stand to be more relaxed (1-Fun) with our feet firmly planted on the ground (2-Shoe); stable, strong, and rooted (3-Tree); more focused (4-Core); more giving (5-Alive); more supported by and connected to our surroundings (6-Thick); more uplifted and inspired (7-Heaven); taking life as it comes to us (8-Gate); pushing back gloomy darkness with a bright sunny disposition (9-Shine) while going with the flow of life (10-Spin). Get the idea?

Before they became mathematics, numerals themselves were considered to be magical. Indeed, the use of numbers in scientific calculations do effect great change in the modern world around us, but ancient man felt that simply drawing them in a proper way would cause beneficial change in the outside world. Now, with the "1 Through 10" Game, they can be magical again as you draw them to create health and wellness within your inner world.

It's almost time for you to pick up your Morning Cup, take a drink, and be a Tai Chi player!

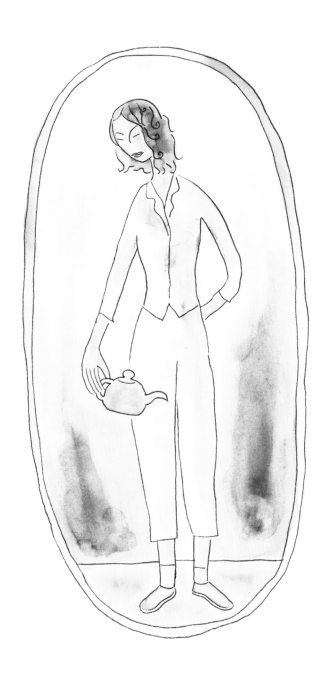

Drawing the Tai Chi Diagram

When you perform your New Forest Tai Chi routine, you will first draw a number (as shown on the preceding pages), then after each number you will draw either a Tai Chi circle, a right-handed Tai Chi diagram, or a left-handed Tai Chi diagram. The Tai Chi diagram, as I described it to you on page 15, is an ancient Chinese symbol from which Tai Chi draws not only its name but its very life force: those powers that work through your muscles and joints to relax and strengthen your body while putting you in touch with your bodymind. What follows are instructions for painting a right-handed Tai Chi diagram. For a left-handed diagram, reverse the right-handed version.

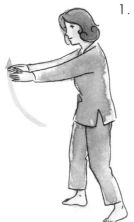

1. Step out on the right foot, hands out in front of you at the bottom of an imaginary circle. Begin to sweep them slowly up and around the left-hand side of the circle.

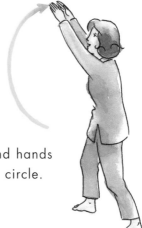

2. Circle your arms and hands up to the top of the circle.

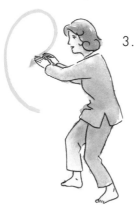

3. When you reach the top of the circle, curve around and down to the right and then back in to the left.

4. When you reach the bottom, sweep your hands and arms up and around to the right, moving counterclockwise.

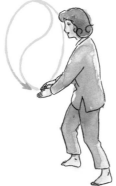

5. Keep going around your circle counterclockwise until you have retraced the entire outer edge of the circle. Stop when your hands reach your starting point at the bottom.

6. This is the right-handed Tai Chi diagram you have just "painted." For a left-handed diagram, step out on the left foot, then move your hands to the right side first.

The Secret of the New Forest

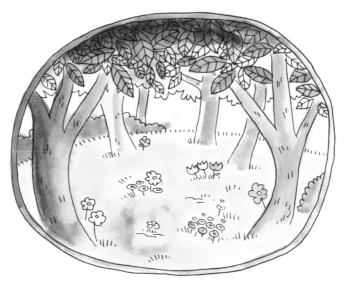

One of the secrets of New Forest Tai Chi is the New Forest itself. To imagine yourself playing Tai Chi in a beautiful, natural setting has a profoundly nourishing effect on your entire bodymind and spirit. The outdoors is, after all, where we take vacations to recharge our batteries. At the turn of the century, physicians regularly prescribed time in nature as a foundation for curing most any illness. Photographs and paintings of nature fill us with awe and inspire us because they remind us of our beginnings. Returning to the forest is a root experience for anyone human.

The Chinese creators of our art used the wonders of the natural world as the primary source of their inspiration for Tai Chi. I've always loved the word "inspired." It means, "in spirit." As you play Tai Chi, you will be playing in the spirit of the natural world, in fact, in the spirit of all creation. While it's always enjoyable to play your Tai Chi outdoors, it is not always convenient or practical. But envisioning the New Forest is something that you can do at any time no matter where you are.

Think of the New Forest as an actual place that exists in a dimension parallel to your everyday world; it's always there, it always has been. You just have to think about it for it to appear. Our Tai Chi forest is a lush, verdant environment teeming with life and energy. Growth and the hidden promise of growth exist all around you. Whatever you need for survival, nourishment, health, and wellness is waiting for you in the New Forest. As soon as you bring this forest into focus, all of the tools and materials needed to be at your best present themselves to you. To my way of thinking, the New Forest represents a return to the Garden, a return to the field of all possibilities where you can rest comfortably in God's hands. This is the ideal place to play your Tai Chi.

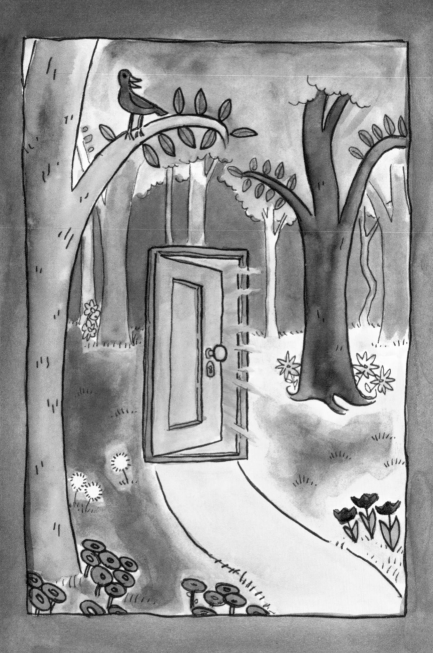

The Routine

Entering the New Forest

It's time for you to enter the New Forest and become a Tai Chi player. Stand with your feet roughly shoulder width apart. At the same time, pretend that a small ball or egg has just appeared under each armpit. This roundness helps your arms, shoulders, and neck to relax. Let your arms hang loosely by your sides. If possible, bend your knees very slightly and only enough to provide you with a feeling of resilience. Let your body be your guide.

Envision the New Forest. Use whatever devices are available to you to imagine it coming into focus: see it, feel it, taste it, and touch it with your imagination. Stand in this posture for a few moments as you silently recite the New Forest keywords: 1-Fun, 2-Shoe, 3-Tree, 4-Core, 5-Alive, 6-Thick, 7-Heaven, 8-Gate, 9-Shine, 10-Spin.

Slowly and deliberately lift both your hands up to shoulder level and just as gently lower them. You are turning on your bodymind so that you can create and shape the postures of Tai Chi.

Now you're ready to begin your Morning Cup routine.

Extra Attention

Some Tai Chi players will stand in this posture for 3-5 minutes, gently cycling through the 10 internal adjustments. This puts them in deeper contact with their bodyminds.

Number 1-Fun

1. Deliberately pick up your right foot and gently step forward and slightly to the right. Step down on your heel and slowly transfer your weight onto it. Keep your hands awake by slightly spreading your fingers, but don't hold them tense or stiffly.

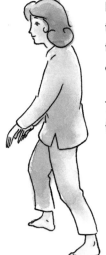

Both feet should be flat on the floor with the knees slightly bent. But don't bend them too much, and try to be as comfortable as you can.

Tai Chi players refer to this kind of forward stepping as a Metal (jin) Step.

2. Bring your hands up and, pretending they are giant paint brushes, paint a big number "1" in the air in front of you.

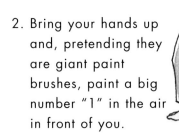

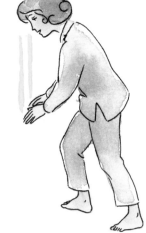

3. When your hands have finished painting the big number "1," start to paint a right-sided Tai Chi diagram.

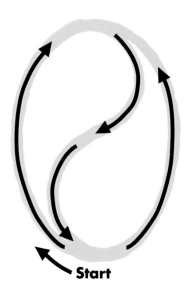

Start

Extra Attention

As you paint the number shape, think "Number 1, the keyword is FUN" and smile faintly. This will help relax your face, head and neck, and shoulders—and it feels good to smile. If it helps, think about something funny.

Inhale as you bring your hands up and exhale as you paint the number. Remember, if at first coordinating the movement with your breath is difficult, just relax and breathe naturally. As you continue to play your Tai Chi, your breath will learn to regulate itself.

You are only as limited as your imagination. See the paint coming from your arms with as much detail as your imagination will allow.

🧍 Number 2-Shoe

1. Take a step forward with your left
   foot, stepping heel-to-toe as you do
   so. Gently lift your hands to the top of
   your imaginary canvas. Breathe!

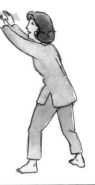

Extra Attention

   At the end of your step, your left leg should bear about 70% of
your body weight, while your right leg holds roughly about 30%.

   Try to remember to keep your left shin perpendicular to the
ground and your feet flat on the floor. This will increase your
overall stability or balance. This is a Tai Chi Metal Step.

2. Slowly paint a
   number "2" shape.
   Inhale as you lift your
   hands, and exhale as
   you paint the number 2.
   Let your waist twist and
   your weight shift as
   much as you want to
   help you make the shape.

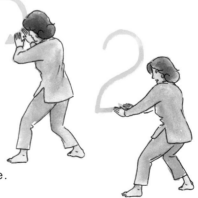

As you paint the number shape, think "Number 2, the keyword is SHOE," and think about your feet and shoes. Pretend that as you are painting the number, you can feel your connection with the earth. You can even suggest to yourself that your toes are squishing their way into warm, muddy soil.

Slow and gentle waist twisting is one of the reasons Tai Chi is such a healthy activity. It's like you're giving your internal organs a healthy massage.

When you twist to the left, Tai Chi players say you are putting Water (shway) in your posture. When you twist gently to the right, you've got Fire (hwo) in it.

3. As soon as you've completed the base of the number "2" shape, lift your hands up and to the right to start your left-sided Tai Chi diagram.

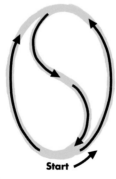

Start

Keep your hands relaxed as you paint the diagram. Remember, if the classic Yin & Yang shape is difficult or confusing, just paint a round Tai Chi circle.

🌳 Number 3 - Tree

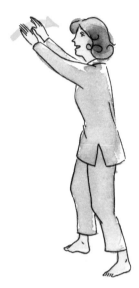

1. Take a forward Tai Chi step with your right foot.

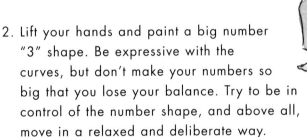

2. Lift your hands and paint a big number "3" shape. Be expressive with the curves, but don't make your numbers so big that you lose your balance. Try to be in control of the number shape, and above all, move in a relaxed and deliberate way.

Extra Attention

As you paint the number, silently say "3-Tree." See yourself as a big sturdy tree with deep roots and strong flexible branches. You can be a tall pine, mighty oak, sturdy hickory, or any kind of tree you want to be. Sway in the breeze to the shape of a big number "3."

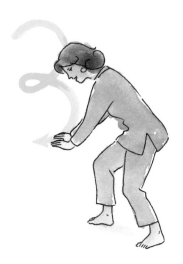

3. Draw a right-sided Tai Chi diagram.

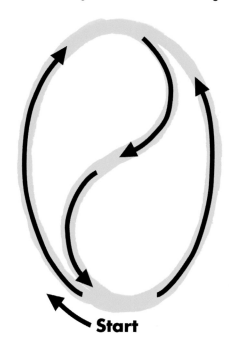

Start

Number 4-Core

1. Pick up your left foot and step down into a stance that is slightly wider than shoulder width. You may place your foot on the ground heel-to-toe or toe-to-heel; you decide.

Extra Attention

Try to evenly distribute your body weight between your feet.

Take as wide a stance as you'd like. Likewise, you can bend your knees a little or a lot. Let your body be your guide.

If you'd like, inhale as you lift up your foot and exhale as you step.

2. With both hands, paint a big number "4" shape on the invisible canvas in front of you. You'll have to lift up your hands at one point to complete the tail of the "4." Be as creative as you are able.

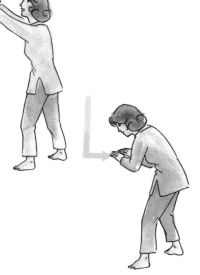

Think "4-Core" as you paint. At the same time, pretend there is a heavy iron fire hydrant resting deep inside your body. Pretend it's heavy and solid, giving you extra weight and stability.

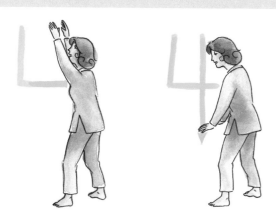

3. Bring your hands up and draw a big Tai Chi circle around the number shape. Let your weight shift from side to side as you draw your circle. Your Tai Chi circle can go to the left or to the right; you decide.

Extra Attention

As you paint your circle, think "4-Core; heavy, solid, sunken, point of focus, I'm strong, I'm sturdy."

Tai Chi players refer to this kind of stepping to a point of central equilibrium as an Earth (tu) step.

Number 5-Alive

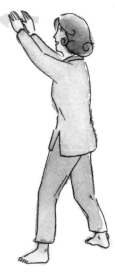

1. Gently step backward with your right foot. If possible, step down toe-to-heel as you shift most of your body weight onto your right leg. In Tai Chi, when you step backward or shift your weight to your rear leg, it is called a Wood (mu) step.

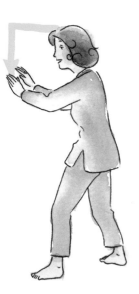

2. Lift your hands and inhale. Place your hands at the top of your invisible canvas and paint a big number "5" shape as you exhale.

Extra Attention

As you paint the number "5" shape, think about water, paint, and energy rushing from your "4-Core" out of your hands and fingers. See it, feel it, taste it, touch it with your imagination. You can even see it coming out of your legs and feet.

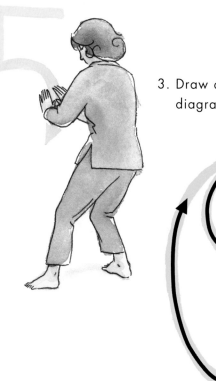

3. Draw a left-sided Tai Chi diagram.

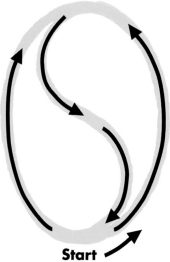

Start

Extra Attention

If possible, inhale as you move up the diagram and exhale as you paint downward.

As usual, you may simply draw a Tai Chi circle if the left-sided diagram is too difficult.

Think about any "5-Alive" idea you can think of as you paint the diagram, such as water rushing out, handshakes, reaching out, or fire hoses.

❄ Number 6-Thick

1. Gently take a mindful step backwards with your left foot. Try stepping down toe-to-heel until the left foot is flat on the ground.

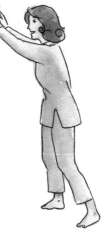

2. Lift your hands in preparation to paint a number "6" shape. Inhale as you lift your hands to the top of your invisible canvas. Paint a flowing, curvy number "6" shape. Be expressive!

Extra Attention

Remember, you can coordinate your breathing with the step. Inhale as you lift your left foot to begin the step and exhale as you put it down. Allow your weight to shift freely back and forth, left and right.

Pretend that the air around you is thick and viscous. It provides slight resistance to your movements as you paint the number "6." Pretend that the thick air that you are moving around in connects you to everything around you (and everyone around you, too).

3. After painting the number "6" shape, flow smoothly into a right-sided Tai Chi diagram.

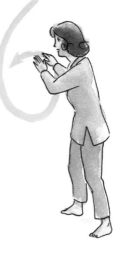

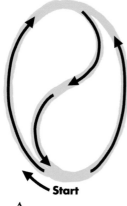

Start

Extra Attention

Whenever possible, inhale as you paint upward on the diagram and exhale as you paint down it.

If you get lost, paint a simple Tai Chi circle on your invisible canvas.

Whether you are painting a full diagram or a simple one, fill your imagination with the idea that the thick air intimately connects you to your immediate surroundings and the people in it. It's as if you were the center of a connective web. Suggest to yourself that if someone or something came into the room where you are playing your Tai Chi you'd be able to feel the web change and vibrate, alerting you to their presence.

Reach out with your imagination to feel the walls (or trees if you're outside) all around you.

Number 7-Heaven

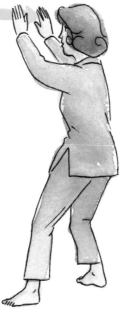

1. Gently shift your weight to your left leg and take a comfortable step backwards with your right.

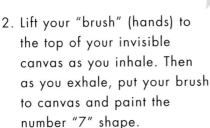

2. Lift your "brush" (hands) to the top of your invisible canvas as you inhale. Then as you exhale, put your brush to canvas and paint the number "7" shape.

Extra Attention

Bend your right knee slightly as if you are about to sit down. Roughly 50 to 60% of your bodymind's weight will rest on it. Remember: you be the judge of what's comfortable for you. Don't bend your knees too much.

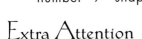

Emphasize the straight lines of the number "7" shape. Particularly, articulate the bend at the top of the "7" shape. For hundreds of years, Tai Chi players have used this maxim when creating their shapes: "Find curves in straight lines and seek straightness in a curve." This is a Tai Chi secret teaching!

As you draw the number "7" shape, pretend that the crown of your head is being gently pulled upward toward heaven, the stars, and all of your higher ideals. It's as if you are a marionette suspended from above.

3. Draw a left-sided Tai Chi diagram. If possible, inhale as you paint upward on your invisible canvas and exhale as you paint downward.

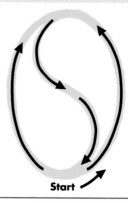

Start

Think of 7-Heaven ideas while painting the Tai Chi diagram: Your hopes, dreams, and wishes; a comforting religious saying; or even a short prayer are all appropriate. It's *important* to think of something that is personally *important* to you. Be as detailed as you'd like and remember to pretend that the crown of your head is being lifted upward toward the heavens. This will generate a light and sensitive feeling, first at the top of your head and eventually over your entire bodymind.

Number 8-Gate

1. Lift your left leg and step down to a stance that is slightly wider than shoulder width. Try to evenly distribute your weight between your feet.

2. Lift your hands upward to the top of the invisible canvas as you inhale. As you exhale, paint the curvy continuous lines of the number "8" shape in one continuous flowing motion. Have fun with this shape!

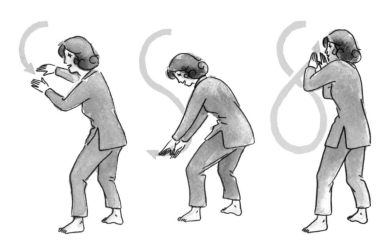

Extra Attention

Take as wide a stance as you are comfortable with. If possible, bend your knees slightly like you're riding a horse or preparing to sit down. How much or how little you bend your knees is up to you. You're in charge.

If you'd like, inhale as you lift your foot and exhale as you set it down. This, like the 4-Core Step, is called an Earth Step ("Tu").

Bend and straighten your knees as much as you want while painting the 8-Gate. Your waist can twist, bend, and turn to accommodate your creativity while painting.

Imagine that you are opening a gate to the energy ebb and flow of life, letting it deeply into your bodymind. Pretend you are successfully navigating the ups and downs of everyday living as you paint. Go with the flow.

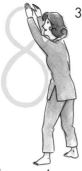

3. Slightly lift your hands off the canvas at the completion of the number "8" shape, then place them back on the invisible canvas and paint a Tai Chi circle around the number "8" shape.

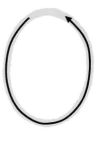

Extra Attention

While playing the circle, exhale as the hands move down the circle and inhale as they paint upward.

Feel free to paint more than one circle. You may even change direction if you like.

Pretend that the pores of your skin are little tiny gates that swing open as you inhale, absorbing the breath of life into your bodymind. When you exhale, imagine that those tiny gates swing closed, trapping life-giving oxygen and healing energy inside of you. While continuing to breathe out, see the air and energy swirling deeply around your muscles and condensing to your bones.

Number 9-Shine

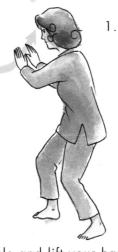

1. Lift your right leg and take a deliberate step forward. If possible, step down heel-to-toe.

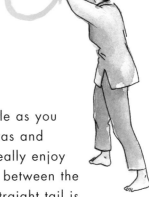

2. Inhale and lift your hands. Exhale as you place them on the invisible canvas and paint the number "9" shape. I really enjoy playing this shape. The contrast between the curvy head of the "9" and the straight tail is fun to create.

Extra Attention

Lift your leg only as high as is comfortable for you. Don't lift so high or step so long that you will lose your balance.

At the end of your right step, try to have roughly 70% of your body weight on your right leg with the remaining 30% on your left leg. Both feet are flat on the ground.

If you coordinate your breathing with your stepping, inhale as you lift your foot and exhale as you put it down.

Whenever you paint this shape, pretend that you are a human light bulb—or even a star, or the sun—that glows brightly, banishing any darkness that happens to be around you.

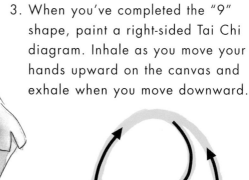

3. When you've completed the "9" shape, paint a right-sided Tai Chi diagram. Inhale as you move your hands upward on the canvas and exhale when you move downward.

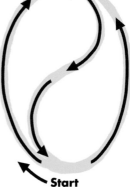

Start

Extra Attention

Think about 9-Shine things while you oscillate through the Tai Chi diagram. For example, during the whole diagram, your bodymind is a bright, shining light bulb that gathers energy as you inhale and shines bright, bright, and brighter still as you exhale.

Nothing pierces gloomy darkness more than the light of surprise and astonishment. See your light illuminating even the farthest corners of your world.

Number 10-Spin

1. Step forward to an even posture with your left foot. If possible, your ending stance should be slightly wider than shoulder width.

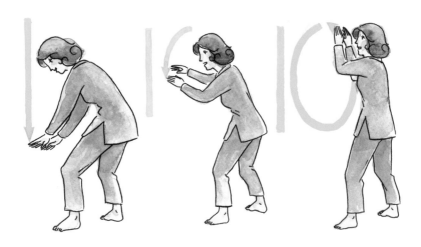

2. You're going to draw two shapes on the canvas: a "1" and a "0" that make up the number "10" shape. Inhale as you lift your hands; exhale and paint the number "1" shape. Then, lift your hands again and paint the "0."

Extra Attention

As in other Earth Steps (4 and 8), bend your knees a little like you're riding a horse or preparing to sit down. The weight of your bodymind is shared evenly between your legs. Feel the earth beneath your feet, which should be flat on the ground.

Remember: if coordinating breath with movements is difficult at first, simply breathe naturally. Your breath will sort itself out on its own as you progress and grow as a New Forest Tai Chi player.

While you are creating the number shape on the invisible canvas, let your mind wander over all the other numbers and keywords and what they mean. It's as if you are a mental juggler, spinning nine dinner plates all at once. Let the numbers and their associated ideas all float and spin inside your imagination.

3. After completing the "0" in your number shape, slightly lift your hands off the canvas and inhale. Place your hands back at the top of the canvas as you exhale and paint the Tai Chi circle around your number "10."

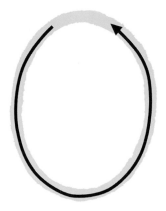

Extra Attention

Continue to let your mind wander over all the numbers "1" through "9" and what they mean to you. If a certain number bubbles up in your imagination more than any other, go ahead and focus on it while painting your simple Tai Chi circle.

Feel free to paint more than one circle during your 10-Spin diagram. Likewise, paint left, right, or change directions as you see fit. After all, it's your Tai Chi!

Leaving the New Forest

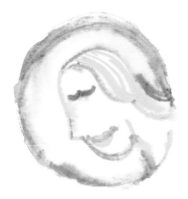

Gently and slowly step in with your right foot to stand with your feet roughly shoulder width apart. Relax your arms, letting them hang naturally to your sides with an imaginary egg under each armpit. If possible, bend your knees just enough to provide a feeling of resilience. Think about the lush, green New Forest and all of the explorations you've done and adventures you've just had. Stand quietly in this posture and review your keywords from 10 to 1: 10-Spin, 9-Shine, 8-Gate, 7-Heaven, 6-Thick, 5-Alive, 4-Core, 3-Tree, 2-Shoe, and 1-Fun.

Slowly and deliberately lift your hands up to shoulder level and just as gently lower them. You are putting your paint, brushes, and canvas away for another time. Then deliberately and gently bring your feet comfortably together and suggest to yourself that having completed your Tai Chi, you are leaving the New Forest to go out and take on your day. In reality, however, the New Forest, with all its secrets and adventures, will always be with you.

Congratulations! You have become a cultivator of life through the art of Tai Chi.

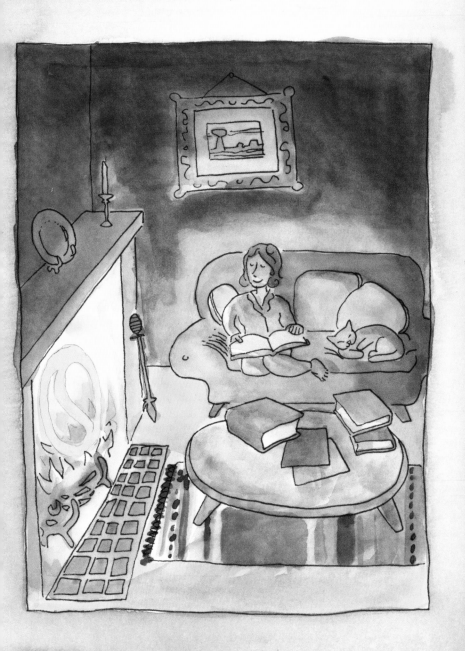

Intermediate Tai Chi Breathing

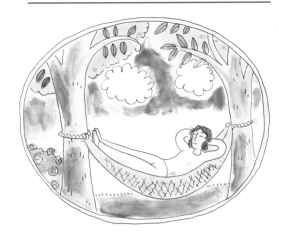

If you are interested in delving deeper into the mysteries of Tai Chi breathing, try the following intermediate exercise. Imagine that there is a balloon in your lower abdomen located about three to five inches below your navel and inward, hidden inside you.

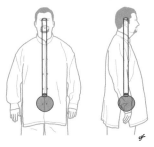

As you breathe in, imagine that the inhaled air goes straight down to this balloon. As you breathe out, imagine that the balloon collapses. Did you notice that I didn't say "contracts as you exhale"? This is very important. You are pretending that the air moves in to and out of your bodymind of its own accord. The air simply comes into your balloon, expanding it to about the size of a grapefruit, and then leaves the balloon, which then collapses as you exhale. Further, imagine that there is a long glass tube that extends from the top of the balloon straight up through the center of your torso and neck. Visualize the opened end of the glass tube pointing upward deep inside the center of your skull. Imagine that the opened end of this tube is where your breathing actually begins. Your nostrils are merely two holes conveniently placed to allow the air you breathe to get to the top of the open glass tube inside your head.

To complete the image, see the air that moves in and out of your bodymind as finely spun silver and gold threads or filaments.

Over time, this way of Tai Chi breathing will change your relationship to precisely how you breathe. Your breath will naturally slow down, and your whole body will relax as your respiration becomes more efficient. Your blood will become filled with life-giving oxygen and energy. This way of breathing is one of the best-kept secrets of Chinese artists, poets, and Tai Chi players. Now, it's yours as well.

As you gain more faculty with your Tai Chi movements, you'll find that you have greater control over your bodymind. Moving very slowly and deliberately will become increasingly more comfortable. "How slow is too slow?" you may ask. My answer is, "suit yourself." If it takes you 5 seconds to paint a number shape or 30 seconds, that's fine. You get to experiment and play. Remember your arms and hands are connected to an inexhaustible supply of paint deep inside of you. If possible, try to begin each shape on an exhalation just like a Chinese calligrapher. Then, as you are completing the number shape or Tai Chi diagram, just breathe naturally without over-focusing.

Traditional Chinese Medicine and Tai Chi

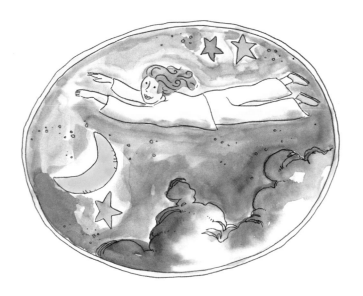

Why is New Forest Tai Chi so good for your health? Because, like other styles of Tai Chi, it is based on the theories of Traditional Chinese Medicine (TCM).

The whole subject of TCM can seem complex and strange to the novice; and rightly so! It would take a lifetime of dedicated study to understand it fully, yet with a little knowledge you can easily understand the fundamental principles of TCM and use them to positively affect your everyday life. New Forest Tai Chi puts this understanding within easy reach.

Qi/Chi ("Life-Force Energy")

Everything has Qi/Chi-life-force energy, including you. Even rocks and cars and air have Qi/Chi. But because you are a living being, you have lots more of it. An abundance of Qi/Chi in your bodymind signifies a robust life while deficient Qi/Chi levels indicate problems. These problems can be emotional, physical, or even intellectual, because your bodymind needs Qi/Chi to do anything from thinking about painting the garage to actually getting around to painting it.

We get a certain amount of Qi/Chi from our mothers at birth. Thereafter we absorb Qi/Chi from our environment, the air we breathe, and the food we eat.

Our Tai Chi is carefully constructed to help us absorb ever-increasing levels of Qi/Chi from our environment and the air we breathe. Furthermore, it moves and distributes this Qi/Chi evenly throughout our bodyminds so that our whole organism can benefit. It even excites the Qi/Chi we already have to higher levels, and we end up bristling with life-force energy.

Popular books on the subject subdivide Qi/Chi into different types, such as Pre-Birth, Post-Birth, and Ancestral Qi/Chi, but these distinctions are not important. All you really need to know is that playing Tai Chi: (1) helps you absorb fresh Qi/Chi from your surroundings and the air you breathe; (2) distributes the fresh Qi/Chi evenly inside you; and (3) excites it to a high level, enlivening your body, your mind, and your spirit.

Ching-Lo: Acupuncture Meridians

The Qi/Chi in your bodymind moves along a specific series of pathways called Ching-Lo, or meridians. These meridians link up and cross-connect all of your organs, bones, and tissues into one coordinated holistic unit. The best way to understand Ching-Lo theory is to think of them as a series of roads and bridges that form an intricate superhighway system. This system—complete with access roads, overpasses, underpasses, rest stops, and weigh stations—is so finely constructed that Qi/Chi in your left pinky toe can travel to your right little finger. If you then think about your bodymind's life-force as the cars and trucks that traverse these roads, then your understanding of Ching-Lo theory is almost complete.

When the traffic on your superhighway system is evenly distributed and flowing smoothly, then you are in a state of ease. But if one of your bridges is being repaired or if there is an accident that is blocking traffic on a stretch of road, then a state of disease exists.

The soft flowing movements of Tai Chi coordinated with breath and imagination repair damaged roads and bridges, clear away accidents and congestion, while directing your inner flow of Qi/Chi to go merrily on its way.

The acupuncturist uses needles and massage to do exactly the same thing, but that's what's so great about Tai Chi—you can do it yourself.

Yin and Yang: Negative and Positive

The words Yin and Yang (or negative and positive) are widely used in TCM in a lot of very different ways. Consequently, it can be confusing. Blood can be too Yin or too Yang. An organ's Yang could be damaged. Too little Qi/Chi is sometimes called Yin and too much sometimes called Yang. Even foods and Chinese herbs can be either Yin or Yang. In truth, two different doctors of TCM will often use these terms in two completely contrary ways.

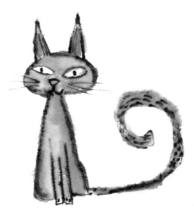

Tai Chi players view the concept of Yin and Yang as the interplay of the two primary forces of life that move through us. It's as if our Tai Chi plays the part of a traffic dispatcher, safely keeping an even number of cars/Yin and trucks/Yang on our superhighway system. If there are too many trucks carrying fuel and food driving in the right side of your bodymind, then the roads can become unsafe for cars. The roads can even wear out prematurely from all the heavy truck traffic. Conversely, if the left side of your bodymind is totally filled with passenger cars then the trucks cannot get to where they are needed. All of the goods and fuel they carry for your bodymind are stuck on the right side of your body.

The weight shifting and soft flowing movements of Tai Chi help keep an equal amount of cars and trucks on your roads, so that the cars can travel safely and the trucks can transport and deliver their goods to the correct destinations.

Some Tai Chi styles emphasize one side of the bodymind over the other and end up damaging the Yin and Yang balance. But not New Forest Tai Chi. The New Forest player steps both forward and backward, twists to the left as well as the right, and uses hand and arm movements that emphasize both the right and left side of the body. In this way, balanced movement on the outside of your bodymind keeps the Yin and Yang balance on the inside of your bodymind as well.

Zhang/Fu: Internal Organs

Everybody knows that a good massage can relax the muscles, ease pain, and free up physical movement. But what about your internal organs? Don't they need to be relaxed and free of pain so they can do their job as well? The answer, of course, is "Yes!"

The waist twisting of New Forest Tai Chi gently massages your guts and viscera, thus encouraging their health and function. Some relatively modern Tai Chi approaches eschew waist twisting in favor of a "Straight back, no bending or twisting" appearance. This is a big mistake. One of the reasons that Tai Chi is so healthy and good for you is because of the way you twist your waist while playing your sequence. When you play Tai Chi, healthy Qi/Chi energy and blood flow are encouraged throughout your organs, just as they are in your arms and legs.

The study of organ function from a TCM perspective is a highly developed and complex issue, but you needn't worry about it at this time. The least you need to know is that twisting the waist while playing Tai Chi will have a beneficial affect on your inner world. And that will affect your outer world, too.

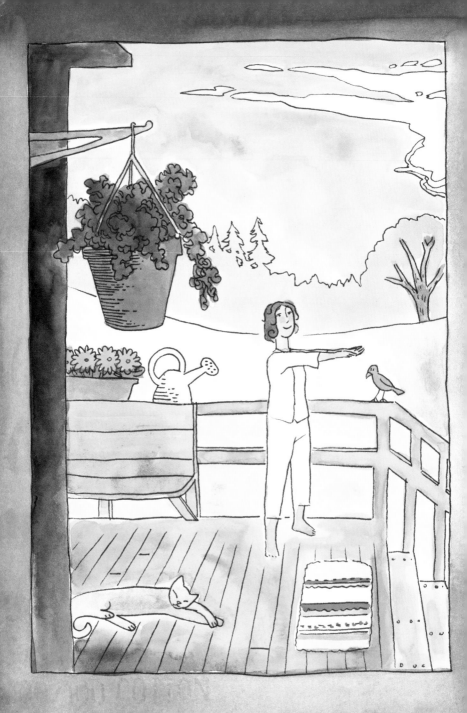

An Extra Sip:
Tai Chi Philosophy

The idea of group classes in Tai Chi is a relatively new concept in the art's history. Chinese people have only been gathering in groups to learn from a Tai Chi teacher since about the 1920s and '30s. Prior to that, instruction took place one-on-one within a strict master-apprentice relationship. This way of transmitting Tai Chi made it necessary for the student to spend long days, weeks, months, and even years practicing alone, perfecting what the master had shown them.

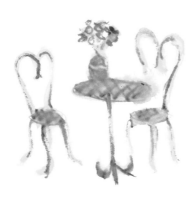

To the Western mind, the idea of practice is to acquire a skill. This is related to our work ethic, which tells us to endure struggle, pain, and hardship now in return for a reward in the future. As the old saying goes, "Practice makes perfect." On the other hand, the ancient Eastern mind regarded practice as a way of creating or revealing the person that is perfect to begin with. To the Tai Chi players of old and the players of today, practice does not make perfect; practice already is perfect.

This unique way of looking at practice makes it necessary for you to have access to sources of inspiration that speak to your artistic sense and stimulate your creativity. Ancient Tai Chi teachers most often recommended the classic Chinese text *The Tao Te Ching*—and so do I.

The Tao Te Ching, more than twenty-three hundred years old, contains so much hidden information about Tai Chi and its practice that you could spend a lifetime pouring over its eighty-one poetic chapters. I've translated four of them for you. Though it's been difficult, I've resisted making any comments about these chapters because I want you to enjoy this extra sip from your Morning Cup alone and in private. I will tell you, however, that if you read them with a Tai Chi mind, you'll find instruction on stepping, breathing, and moving. There are clues about how to create and play. There are even secrets about how to live a fuller life. I hope you'll find them helpful as you continue your life as a player of Tai Chi. Enjoy!

Selected Chapters from the Tao Te Ching

Chapter Eight

if a person wants to be at their best
then they should pattern themselves after water

water serves the land and the life on the land

it gives this life by moving through the land
seeking its own balance and equilibrium

this is in contrast to human beings who always look up
and think of rising to some lofty achievement

water will always flow around obstacles
and seek out the lowest earthbound space and opening that it can
find

in this way
it is always closer to the miracle of life than we are

the miracle talks to us through water

and it says

wherever you choose to live remember
the earth beneath your feet
consider how to feel it with all that you do

whenever you want peace remember
to flow into your heart and mind
plunging into the profound love that resides deep within you

however difficult remember
that you should speak frankly
but never drown others with your words

whichever instances call for leadership remember
that a constant stream helps order
the life around it

whatever business you transact remember
to go steadily to the source
and dutifully perform without washing up on unprepared land

if you listen to me
when there is a call to action
the miracle will tell you when it is time to act

contending causes contention

have no part of it
and you will be a cool stream
that is nourishing to all

Chapter Twelve

imagine a soft light of bluegreen
imagine a strong red light
imagine a rich yellow light
imagine a bright white light
now imagine the black absence of color

if you look at these lights singly you will know what they are

if you allow them into your eyes all at once
then you will not be able to distinguish one from the other

the twelve musical notes can be arranged magically to create a
joyful noise

the twelve musical notes can also be thrown together without
method
like stones in a hole
that becomes an ordinary activity that denies the hole its usefulness

attempt to
eat something sour
eat something bitter
eat something sweet
eat something pungent
eat something salty
all at the same time and the once pleasant tastes are likely to
nauseate you

ordinary people exceed the basic goodness of the things of this
world
in searching for new ways to exceed themselves

the momentum of exceeding unbalances the heart and mind
and generates insecurity and a loose footing that denies the true
self

for these reasons
the sound person speaks to the unconscious heart and mind
requesting instructions on how to nourish the true self

when gently asked
the unconscious teaches appreciation for those things that are
within us all

when gently asked
the unconscious teaches circumspection for those things that are
without us all

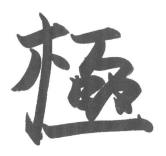

Chapter Sixteen

deliver all your inner confusion to the earth
and resting quietly
leave your mind undisturbed

allow all things that manifest and their roots
to assume definite shape
and move about in activity
against the backdrop of your reflective awareness
and observe these events passively with a controlled heart and
simple spirit

when these bustling shapes slow down and cease in their activity
and return to the nothingness from whence they came
you will attain a state of quietude
that is an imitation of the tao way of life
without force it occurs naturally
and is called ceaseless and faithful
it is known as the law of mundane transposition
in this state you will see yourself as you truly are
this perspective must shock you a little
or it will not be genuine as a picture of your true self

understanding this law of mundane transposition
begets tolerance of self and others

understanding tolerance of self and others
begets wisdom of self and others

understanding the wisdom of self and others
begets infinite insight into self and others

employing the insight of self and others creates resonance with
the heavens
the earth
and man

employing this resonance
creates an alignment with the tao way of life

thus aligned you will directly communicate with the miracle
and even in ordinary death will forever be a part of it

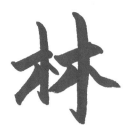

Chapter Twenty-Two

bend the waist	as pliable yellow gold
flex the joints	in the shape of metal
twist the limbs	as a tree

integral growth

make yourself an empty vessel
and receive the chi life force of the universal

see yourself as deep and vast
yet softly muted to the ordinary world

standing alone under the sky
this firmament over your accepted perceptions

is perpetual renewal in which the smallest piece of wealth

is a vast natural fortune
that will go unnoticed
unless the heavens are above your head

this message is so utterly simple
that it is easily confused by over-thinking

when heaven is in your head
rather than above it
you will be scattered into space
without a home

but when heaven is in its place in the sky
real comprehension and
conscious comprehension
remain fixed to the core center in balance

then
you have returned home

an insightful person embraces and holds the absolute
singularity reflected as the original mind
consuming the consummate

and the absolute becomes a limitless model
of plenary usage

containing all possibilities
of all that is possible

remain esoteric and invite wisdom
deny light to ordinary eyes
and sound to ordinary ears

in order to balance the mind and clear perception

though this ongoing quest is a personal endeavor
refrain from forcing life to be about yourself

do not force the hearts and spirits of others
in self-gratification
for this damages your vitality and essence

denial of accolades from yourself and others
to yourself
is a way to balance the conscious ordinary comprehension with real
comprehension

in this way the ordinary world
will be at peace with you
and you with it

all of this requires you to remain adaptable
to the ever-changing present

bend   flex   twist
pliable gold shaping metal living tree

yes
surely these are watchwords

that preserve the integral gifts of human existence

in that
they belong to all

Tai Chi and Chinese Calligraphy

represents clouds in a blue sky.

is the picture of a
dragon in that sky.

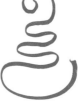

shows the force of a thunderstorm.

Tai Chi postures have their roots in ritual Taoist movement. In the ancient Taoist tradition, this movement is taught through the practice of mystic brush writing known as "Celestial Calligraphy." Taoist adepts first learn their magical gestures by writing on paper (either yellow or white), or on a special table covered with fine red sand, or on the surface of a large bowl of water. Their implements are brush and hand-ground red or black ink, a twig made of peach or willow wood, or the hands and fingers held in arcane formations. These implements hold immense significance.

But it is the mystic characters themselves—and the way they are taught—that concern us in this historical discussion of Meaningful Shapes. First, the Tai Chi teacher draws the character on a piece of paper. The student then copies the master's work, attempting to capture the same essence in his own creation. The master corrects the student's work by adjusting the student's posture and grip on the writing implement. He instructs the student in the use of specific visualizations for each stroke of the celestial character and for the character as a whole. More detailed instruction in the form of verse is recited by the master. Repeated drawings and corrections continue until the master and the student become rhythmically entrained in a mystic flow of artistic call and response. Eventually, the heart of the celestial character is fully transmitted to the fledgling calligrapher.

These characters and thousands more—having been learned and executed with brush and ink—become, on a larger scale, movements of the entire bodymind. They must be drawn in the air with all requisite intent, inner dynamics, and history—and as much meaning as the mystic artist can bring to it.

The ancient creators of Tai Chi believed that number shapes contained and supported distinctive symbolism and importance. As New Forest players, we regard our number shapes with the very same importance.

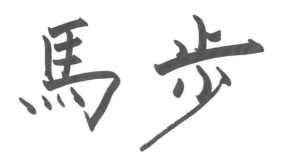

About the Author

John Bright-Fey is a 40-year veteran of the Chinese Health Exercise and Martial Arts. A highly accomplished Master Instructor, he is an expert and world-renowned authority on Tai Chi.

John moved to Alabama from California in 1990 with his wife, Kim, a licensed physical therapist and certified Kung-Fu instructor. A year later, he opened the Blue Dragon Academy in Hoover, Alabama, where he teaches Tai Chi and other Chinese disciplines.

His instructional video "New Forest Tai Chi for Beginners" consistently ranks among the top-selling videos in the country.

The Routine at a Glance

Number 1-Fun

Number 2-Shoe

Number 3-Tree

Number 4-Core

Number 5-Alive

Number 6-Thick

Number 7-Heaven

Number 8-Gate

Number 9-Shine

Number 10-Spin

Tear this page out and post it on your refrigerator or another handy spot for quick reference to your Tai Chi routine.

If you would like to learn more about Tai Chi, visit the author's website, www.newforestway.com, featuring the video "New Forest Tai Chi for Beginners."